A Better Normal for Changes in Erection

Your Guide to Rediscovering Intimacy After Cancer

Tess Devèze

Published in Australia by ConnectAble Therapies Pty Ltd.

1510 Mills Road, Glen Forrest WA 6071, Australia
Copyright © 2023 Tess Devèze
All rights reserved.

Disclaimer: All care has been taken in the preparation of the
information herein, but no responsibility can be accepted by the author
for any damages resulting from the misinterpretation of this work. The
content in this book shall not be used as an alternative to seeking
professional and clinical advice.

For more information see www.connectabletherapies.com

ISBN: 978-0-6458244-0-7

CONTENTS

WHY I WROTE THIS BOOK

Hello! It's so wonderful to meet you. I'm Tess.

I thought before we get into the more 'intimate' details, I'd introduce myself and let you know what this book is about.

I was diagnosed with stage-three breast cancer in 2018, at the age of 36. At the time of my diagnosis, I'd been working in the sexuality sector for years. Over the years since my cancer diagnosis and endless treatments, only twice did a healthcare professional voluntarily bring up the topic of sexuality and only one booklet was recommended to me (which I had to go and find myself). The lack of information and support on this topic, both during and after treatments, was painfully noticeable.

Why aren't more resources available? Why are we so afraid to talk about this essential aspect of our lives?

First and foremost, I'm an occupational therapist (OT). What's an OT, I hear you ask? We are functional therapists and use specific approaches to promote independence and participation in 'occupations' which are any kind of meaningful life activity that occupies us. OT's help you do the day-to-day activities that you need and want to do, as best you can. This may include self-care tasks (shower, dressing, toileting), work related (vocational) tasks, social or community activities…and may also include sex!

My clinical experience is mostly in sexuality - during and after cancer treatments, brain-injury, neurological conditions, and those living with disability. Before moving solely to sexuality for people with cancer, disability and chronic illness, most of my work was in private and public hospitals across Australia, working in neurological rehabilitation. I love neuroscience, and most of my work is based on neurological concepts.

Other than having cancer and being a sexuality OT, I also work with sexuality and self-development pioneers 'Curious Creatures', based in Melbourne Australia. I've facilitated hundreds of workshops online and face to face for nearing a decade, teaching consent, better intimacy and communication skills. I've seen thousands of people's lives change through a deeper understanding of sexual intimacy.

Lastly, I've also studied somatic sexological bodywork at the Institute of Somatic Sexology. This training has given me a deeper understanding of how libido, pleasure, arousal and orgasmicity (cool word huh?) work on a physiological, neurological, and psychological level. These learnings form an essential part of this book.

Even with all my training, I've struggled. If you're struggling too, you're not alone (even if it doesn't get spoken about).

But it's not just about me. The contents of this book are also guided by you. I have a Facebook group 'Intimacy and Cancer' with thousands of people - all cancers, all genders - from over 49 countries, who share and support each other on this topic. My one-on-one clients have also been a huge source of learning, generously sharing their experiences.

It's been almost two years since releasing 'A Better Normal; Your Guide to Rediscovering Intimacy After Cancer', and the positive feedback I have personally been receiving from readers has been at times overwhelming. I am humbled, amazed and inspired by the impact and influence this book has had for those out there suffering.

But cancer treatments are *haaaaaard*, and so is reading! I wanted to know how I could reach more people, change more lives for the better through the contents in this book. In answer to that question, I've created the 'A Better Normal' mini-book *series*. It's a number of bite-sized treatment or side-effect specific mini-books, to help cancer patients and their loved ones maintain and grow connection, intimacy and sexuality. Each mini-book is created from the information in 'A Better Normal; Your Guide to Rediscovering Intimacy After Cancer', but broken down into simple, easy-to-read guides relative to your very specific needs, because often during and after treatments committing to a 300-page book feels overwhelming or is simply not possible.

Books in the 'A Better Normal' mini-book series are:

- 'A Better Normal for **Libido**; Your Guide to Rediscovering Intimacy After Cancer'
- 'A Better Normal for **Vaginal Dryness & Pain**; Your Guide to Rediscovering Intimacy After Cancer'
- 'A Better Normal for **Body Confidence**; Your Guide to Rediscovering Intimacy After Cancer'
- 'A Better Normal for **Chemotherapy**; Your Guide to Rediscovering Intimacy After Cancer'
- 'A Better Normal for **Hormone Therapy**; Your Guide to Rediscovering Intimacy After Cancer'
- 'A Better Normal for **Fatigue**; Your Guide to Rediscovering Intimacy After Cancer'

- 'A Better Normal for **Changes In Erection**; Your Guide to Rediscovering Intimacy After Cancer'
- 'A Better Normal for **Radiotherapy**; Your Guide to Rediscovering Intimacy After Cancer'
- 'A Better Normal for **Pain**; Your Guide to Rediscovering Intimacy After Cancer'

Or if you're after all of the above information (and more) in one place, the all-in-one book 'A Better Normal; Your Guide to Rediscovering Intimacy After Cancer' has everything you need.

If you end up with several mini-books in the series, that's pretty normal, as we don't have only one side-effect (geez, wouldn't that be nice!), and we can have the same side-effect from more than one treatment (like fatigue, or changes in libido). Cancer treatments impact us differently, which is why some books in this series are side-effect specific, and others treatment specific. So you can pick and choose what is most relevant for you and where you're at. You'll also notice that some mini-books have repeated information in them. That's because some information is essential and helpful, regardless of what your side-effect or treatment is (like the communication tips, or ways to gently reconnect with yourself or a partner).

The most important thing you can learn from this book is that you're not alone and you're not broken. There's nothing wrong with you if you're struggling. It's normal to find this situation tough. This isn't one-size-fits-all advice. All bodies are unique, every relationship is different, and everyone experiences relationships, connection, pleasure and desire in their own way. You're the expert on you! Just as cancer is different for everyone, so are the connections we have with ourselves and those around us.

Lastly, this book is for all human beings, regardless of gender, lifestyle, orientation, ability, ethnicity, age, or relationship dynamic. Although every person with cancer is unique, we have one thing in common: no matter who we are or what we are going through, we're all worthy of love and connection.

Now, let's get started on making your 'new normal', a 'better normal'.

1.   KEY TERMS EXPLAINED

Sexuality vs sex

The word 'sexuality' is an umbrella term which yes includes the functional activity of sex, but also includes relationships, connections, affection, dating, pleasure and our overall well-being. Sexuality can be greatly affected due to cancer, but it doesn't necessarily have to stop altogether. As a sexuality educator and clinician, I know how important sexuality, connection and intimacy is to our quality of life, our resilience and coping. What could be more important!

'Sex' in this book refers to the act, or the activity you engage in with yourself and/others, and is one of the most diverse and most adaptable functional activities I can think of. Yet today, it's still one of the most under-addressed topics in clinical settings. This is something I aim to change.

I also want us all to be on the same page in how we see 'sex' itself which is more than just orgasms and genital play, it's so much more. During cancer treatments and other life-altering events, you might need to temporarily let go of traditional forms of touch/sex. We can become excited, aroused, release pleasure hormones in our body from so many different ways. There are erogenous zones all over our bodies such as our inner thighs, breasts, nipples, under the armpits, the neck, earlobes, feet and many more depending on your body. Orgasms, engorgement, ejaculation, becoming 'hard' or 'wet', these don't need to be your goal, but can also be experienced in more than one way. Pleasure, enjoyment, arousal, excitation and connection, that is where the fun can also be. Pleasure is pleasurable and our whole body can be pleasured!

Desire vs arousal

Desire (the wanting) I use interchangeably with libido. Desire/libido are the experience of *wanting* sex and pleasure. Desire has many words that can be used, such as lust, sex-drive, and essentially all refer to that *want* we have.

Arousal is the way our body responds when it's in pleasure, the changes in our body that show us we are in fact, enjoying and excited. Things like increased sensitivity, maybe we become wet, maybe we become hard, our heart rate increases, we breathe heavier and more.

Simply put, libido = wanting, and arousal = enjoying.

Treatments can affect our arousal as well as our libido, which I dive into in this book, but knowing the difference between these can be very helpful.

The magical word, intimacy

Disconnection from yourself and others is a common side-effect of cancer treatments for so many. You're not alone in this and here I introduce you to the magical word 'intimacy'. Imagine that you having sex or being intimate again with yourself, a date or a partner/s, is the goal or the prize. That prize is on the other side of a river, and to get to it, you need to build a bridge. How can you do that? Through intimacy, through touch and the other magical word *affection*.

I've heard many times from clients and people in my support group "we don't even touch each other anymore". Not only has sex gone, but so has the *intimacy*, and are we really going to want sex without that connection?

Intimacy and affection are small giants. Tiny little things that can mean the world, and build that bridge of connection. Things like hand-holding, a good-night kiss, a good morning hug, your arm around your partner in the kitchen, cuddling on the couch, touch for the sake of touch (not as a way to 'get somewhere'), massage swaps, maybe a cheeky butt-squeeze and grin, and the big one, WORDS OF LOVE.

When you want some touch or love? Here's a few ways to ask, without that pressure of it needing to lead to sex:

How to say it out loud.

- "Hey, I'd like to be closer to you, how about a cuddle?"
- "Can we snuggle together on the couch while watching this film?"
- "You up for some hand-holding while we walk to the shop?"
- "I'm loving you right now, thought I'd share."
- "You up for some underwear-on cuddling while we fall asleep? I miss connecting with you."
- "I'd love some touch/to touch your body, would you like a massage?"
- "I'm not wanting this to lead to sex, but some kisses and cuddles would be lovely if you're feeling like some connection?"
- "I'm checking you out right now, just wanted to share."

- "I'm running a bath to relax and wind-down from the day, would you like to join me for some down-time?"

Small giant steps towards that prize.

2. COMMUNICATING'S HARD, BUT IMPORTANT

Please don't be down on yourself if you're struggling (whether you're a partner or the person diagnosed). Things are hard, things are different. It's okay, there are workarounds (which I'll get into soon). Ignore external pressures and expectations and focus on yourself and each other. Not only do our bodies and lives change from cancer, so do our roles. From partner to patient, lover to carer, friend to carer etc. You can get through it, together.

Silence is the enemy and can be common when we're finding things difficult. Fear and uncertainty are prevalent during treatments and we can withdraw from each other intentionally or unintentionally. It makes sense that we don't talk about the thing that's hard to talk about!

Fear of dating, meeting new people, of hurting a partner, not knowing how their/your new body works or not wanting to cause pain can all be reasons someone withdraws. Plus, your partner/loved one has seen you go through one of the hardest things of your life, be more unwell than ever, it's scary stuff.

For reasons above and more, not knowing how to

interact and pulling away is common.

For the people with the diagnosis, understanding what is happening in our body and communicating that? That can feel impossible. Either way, humans have not evolved to read minds, so you'll need to break the silence and share what's happening. So often, the concerns we have in our minds seem a lot bigger when they stay in our minds. Talking is key.

And while we're at it, please don't compare yourself to anyone else or any other relationships. It's the fastest way to unhappiness at any level and that includes comparing yourself to yourself, the 'pre-cancer you'. I call myself 'Tess BC' (BC = before cancer) when I'm in that loop. I often think of my pre-cancer body and mind, how I used to have less pain, more energy, body parts that used to be there, how I could remember things and focus on tasks, so you're not alone in this. I constantly remind myself, comparisons to others or the way things used to be won't change anything. It's such an easy pattern to fall into. I'm sorry to be so blunt as it's hard not to think about what has changed and how things used to be, but please try to think ahead. Cancer is different for everyone and every relationship is different.

There are millions of us fighting cancer, with suffering sexuality. It can be scary, but you don't have to do this alone.

Who to ask and how to ask

Communication with your loved ones isn't the only thing that's essential, but also communication with your treating team. Knowing who to ask about sexuality, positioning, care & *safety* is something most of us don't know.

Here's a general summary.

Gynaecologists work with people who have a vulva and/or vagina. Urologists work with those who have a penis. Gastroenterologists and colorectal surgeons work with the digestive system including bowel cancers. Haematologists work with blood and lymphatic cancers. You will also have medical professionals relative to your treatments such as a radiation oncologist for radiotherapy treatments, an endocrinologist for hormone treatments and the effects they have on our bodies and sexuality, and your oncologist who oversees your treatments. You will have a surgical team relative to the type of procedure you will be having. Psychiatrists are who to speak with regarding mental health and medications, including which medications have which impacts on your sexuality.

All of these people plus your nurses, your doctor or GP (general practitioner if you're in Australia) are all trained to answer your questions.

There are also people like me (OT's) who focus on sexuality, there's pelvic floor physiotherapists and OT's, there are sexologists and sex counsellors as well. You will need to ask; you will need to be your own advocate for your sexuality. But don't worry, if they're not sure how to best answer your question, they will find someone who is. Your care is their priority.

I hear you saying "sure Tess, it's easy to tell us to ask medical professionals questions, but *how* do you ask the questions?" The first step (asking) is the hardest…. But you can do it, I've got your back!

How to say it out loud.

- "What are the precautions I need to take regarding sexual activities during this treatment?"
- "Do I need to avoid sex or do specific things safety-wise? If so, when and for how long?"
- "What do I and my partner/s need to know or do

regarding intimate activities?"

- "I'd like to ask a few questions about sex and intimacy during and after my treatments. Is there a more private space we could go to?"

- "Is there someone I can speak with, who can answer questions about sex during and after treatment?"

- "We/I would like to discuss intimacy during/after treatment. Can we organise a time? And with who?"

- "I'm experiencing some changes with my (insert issue here). Who is the best person to speak to? "

- "How will this treatment affect me/us intimately? "

- "Are there any potential sexual side-effects I should be aware of?"

- "I'm not sure how to ask this, but I have some questions of a more private nature, who can I speak with about that?"

If a healthcare professional isn't sure or cannot answer your question?

- "Thanks for letting me know, can you please ask someone who might be able to answer?"

- "Okay, can you please tell me who I can ask?"

3. CHANGES IN ERECTION

As a sexual organ that is mostly on the outside of the human body and highly visible, changes in penis function can cause a lot of body-shame and anxiety.

I must say that your penis is capable of extreme pleasure without needing to be hard or erect. Orgasms are entirely possible, even if you cannot be erect or ejaculate.

For people who are experiencing changes in function, the resource 'A Touchy Subject' is run by a clinical sexuality and prostate cancer researcher Victoria Cullen. She specialises in penile and sexual health post prostatectomy. Victoria offers a broad range of information that is relevant for anyone and everyone with erectile challenges and her work is changing lives for the better. Her website includes free erectile recovery programs via email, an info YouTube channel (search 'A Touchy Subject'), written articles and clinical discussions and reviews for items such as pumps and vacuum devices.

Another powerful tool, for anyone with a penis experiencing changes in erection, but also loss of sensitivity, pleasure and orgasm, is soft penis massage. Not only is a soft penis capable of pleasure and orgasm, but offering yourself (or a partner giving you) regular massage increases blood-flow and sensation. If done regularly it can have benefits such as recovering orgasms, increasing sensitivity and for some, erectile recovery. I've supported many folks (including post-prostatectomy) learn soft penis massage and it's had pretty amazing pleasure and erectile outcomes. The most effective way to get results is to do it regularly (a few times a week is great), because of course, it's about neurologically rewiring pleasure and function. Take a look at the 'Penis Pleasure Masterclass' info in the 'resources' section at the end of this book for more information.

Something very important. If you're in the process of recovering your erectile function and health, know it takes time. Years. You might hear someone say "3 months to 2 years", but that three-month figure is very, *very* rare. Please see this as long-term and keep at it. It is normal to not see much change in the first year, nerve repair takes a *minimum* of six months. I only say this to manage expectations and avoid disappointment, shame, and the potential to give up. This is a long-haul process, but recovery is possible, it does take time (but in the meantime, you always have injections, so please chat to your urologist, radiation oncologist or doctor about them!).

There are many options such as; penile massage for neural rehab, Viagra (which doesn't always work), pumps and vacuum devices (the 'vacurect' is having absolutely amazing results for users), medications, injections (needles are nerve-wracking, but are a wonderful option for you!) physical rehabilitation, pelvic floor work and toys (refer to the 'it's toy time' section coming up). There's also a podcast called 'The Penis Project' hosted by a men's-health physiotherapist and a sexologist/nurse practitioner. They share so much information on erectile and continence recovery through interviewing everyday people, and sharing their own professional advice. They really know their stuff! You don't need to do this alone and your urologist, physiotherapist, oncologist, radiation oncologist, doctor, Victoria Cullen, The Penis Project and I, are all here for you.

Something that does need to be given voice, is the shame we can feel from changes in our sexual function. Our culture has told many of us that a hard penis means enjoyment, an erect penis means that things are 'going well'. Soft penises to some are regarded as non-sexual, that a person needs to 'try harder to get hard' or a soft-cock means that they don't find you attractive or don't want to be intimate with you. As the penis is on the outside of the human body, whether you're soft or hard, it's hard to hide. You're exposed and so is your 'arousal'. I feel for you, and I'm so truly sorry if you have ever experienced shame due to your delightful, sensual, soft-penis.

News flash everyone: a soft penis is delicious, sensitive and can still experience pleasure. As the giver of sexual touch to a soft penis, it can be (and is) extremely pleasurable to offer pleasure and play, without things needing to be hard or erect. Plus, it's also very enjoyable for the receiver. You can orgasm without an erection and you can orgasm without a prostate gland if you don't have one. I say this as someone who coaches people post prostatectomy (prostate removal) on exactly this. How to experience pleasure and orgasm with a soft-penis and rehabilitate function (refer to the 'Penis Pleasure Masterclass' in the 'resources' section for more on that).

To anyone that has seen a soft penis and said out loud or thought in their head "what's wrong?", please, please, don't think this way. The pressure of getting erect can be one of the things that interferes with the process of getting erect. After surgeries, medications, chemo, stress, fatigue & pain, getting erect may be difficult. Please understand, soft-penises are wonderful, sexy and still capable of pleasure.

Of course, if there are ongoing issues, consult your doctor, but being hard doesn't mean you're 'good' at sex, for the giver or for the receiver. Being good at sex isn't about how hard you get, or how hard you make someone else get, it's about how you touch, communicate, offer and enjoy pleasure.

Exercise

There is a *lot* of research and evidence that connects exercise with erectile health. Please do not think I'm saying that if you go for a jog every day, your erections will be magically recovered. However, regular exercise can have positive influences on your erectile health and also, erectile recovery (this includes people post prostate cancer treatments). Cardiovascular exercise (exercise that gets your heart rate up) promotes blood-flow and vascular health. With healthy blood vessels and regular circulation (through exercise), not only does your circulation improve, the tissues can also become healthier. Additionally, regular physical activity can help some people be more receptive to erectile drugs.

Depending on your treatment history, physical and cardiovascular status, you will need to be careful. I'm not going to make a specific exercise regime recommendation here as people can experience changes in erection for varied reasons, and we all have different bodies. So, you will need an exercise routine that is relevant for you, provided by a medical professional who knows you. It's vital you talk to your treating team/a medical professional who knows your treatment history and current level of physicality, so you can incorporate cardiovascular health and exercise into your erectile health routine s*afely* and *effectively.*

4. CHANGES IN SENSATION

I've been speaking quite generally about how we can rehabilitate our desire and strengthen our pleasure pathways, but I'm going to get a little more specific in this section. In particular, the permanent loss of sensation and erogenous zones through surgeries & treatments, and how losing sensation doesn't necessarily mean losing your sexuality.

The amazing thing about the human body is that we can create *new* erogenous zones! Remember, our sex and pleasure are what's between our ears and not our legs.

If you're experiencing a loss of sensation due to the removal of a part of your body which would include nerve removal, or your treatments have damaged the nerves, sensation in this particular part of your body may or may not ever come back. But there is hope.

Sensation where nerves are intact is exactly the same as a bicep that gets stronger as you exercise it. You can 'create' and 'recreate' highly pleasurable erogenous zones all over (and in) your body, with slow soft touch and being present to how good it feels. In particular, if you're feeling numbness and loss of sensation on or in your genitals, repeated touch and in particular massage can 100% help you regain your sensation and pleasure (refer to the 'Penis Pleasure Masterclass' information in the 'resources' section). If you have loss of sensation due to permanent nerve damage or removal, over time, you can have such amazing pleasure from other areas of your body (neck/inner thighs/ears/lips/belly/lower back etc.). How is this done?

Being intimate, focussing on *slow touch* while being curious can start the rewiring process. It's how we create new erogenous zones and enhance pleasure/sensation that may already be there, but just isn't very strong. If you're wanting to recover sensation and pleasure on/in your genitals, I can't recommend soft penis massage highly enough. Even just twice a week has great outcomes over time.

If you're wanting to recover and improve sensation on your body, play the 2-minute game (described in the section 'simple ideas for connecting') asking for attention to other parts of your body, offer yourself soft slow touch when you wake up in the morning for 5 minutes each day or if you need extra support and guidance, my online 'connection & cancer' course (detailed in the 'resources' section). Your inner thighs can be just as erotic as say, your breasts once were with touch.

I've used the same techniques to help people post-stroke regain sensation on their arms, when working in neurological rehabilitation. With a little repetition and attention, you can enhance your pleasure and sensitivity too. Neurological change doesn't happen overnight, but over time it can and does happen.

Remember, pleasure is still pleasurable, even if it's somewhere else on your fabulous body.

In the meantime, brain-chatter from things like self-consciousness, anxiety or stress can be the barrier to enjoying touch on your body and also that rewiring process. If you're getting intimate and feeling self-conscious about your body, pop an item of clothing that's a lovely, sensual material. Something that *feels* nice and helps reduce anxiety. This will help get your head back into the experience.

It's okay to get sexy while wearing clothing. Or try some positions that aren't so full-frontal to help you relax and enjoy (like the spoon/side-lying position, or from behind). The key to enhancing your pleasure, to strengthening those sensory and pleasure pathways is to be present, and we can't do that when we're in our heads.

I also want to note as someone who has lost sensation on a large part of my body from surgeries and treatments, that I have a sense of loss. Loss of a part of my body which was a source of *so* much pleasure for me. Please allow yourself time to grieve, process and share how you're feeling. None of this is easy, but the loss of a body part, or loss of sensation on an area of your body doesn't have to mean the loss of your sex or your pleasure all together.

Just like everything else in cancer, it's a process and can take time, but speaking from personal experience as someone who has rehabilitated themself through these touch and massage practices, it's well worth it.

5. REACTIVE AROUSAL VERSUS PROACTIVE AROUSAL

I'd like to discuss arousal responses for a moment. Remember, arousal is the way our body responds *in* pleasure, our enjoyment. Libido is the wanting and desire. As discussed earlier in this book, arousal responses could include things like an increase in heart rate, our pupils dilate, skin sensitivity increases, erection, tissues become engorged, we become wet, we become hard and more.

Delayed arousal responses are extremely common from treatments and medications, and can also be caused by many psychological aspects like stress and nervousness. Just like we have the many layers (physiological, psychological and neurological) that can impact our libido, so do these layers potentially impact our arousal. What this can look like, is you don't 'want it as much' (or at all), it takes a lot longer for you to 'get into it' than it used too. That you notice it feels like maybe you're forcing yourself at the start, but after some time, things start to feel more enjoyable. Sound familiar?

I call this **'reactive** vs **proactive'** pleasure and arousal.

Reactive means, in *response* to something. You *react* to a thing or stimulus. With arousal and pleasure, that could look like only feeling aroused *after* you have been kissing and touching for some time. You're reacting to the touch and intimacy.

Proactive means something that happens *without* prompt or stimulus. It happens without needing something to react too. In pleasure and arousal this could look like you're watching television and all of a sudden, you're gagging for it. Or you walk down the street enjoying the sun on your face and you then notice your underwear is damp and the breeze feels soooo good!

Countless people feel their enjoyment of sex is gone forever, that they have lost their desire completely because their pleasure and arousal seem now absent (is no longer proactive). But in actual fact, it's just now more reactive and it needs something to respond to. It needs a bit more pleasure time to kick in. There's a gigantic difference between someone who doesn't enjoy sex at all versus someone who needs time to enjoy it.

I support many who think they cannot stand sex at all anymore and are desperate to reclaim this part of their life, and when I ask "So what do you do to warm-up before sex?" This question is followed by silence, a tumbleweed rolls past and that's the moment where I get my whiteboard out.

I'd like you (and anyone you're with) to grab a piece of paper and a pen, a notebook, or anything you can individually draw and write on. Now, draw a very basic XY graph (just a small graph is fine) with the Y axis labelled as 'arousal' and the X axis labelled as 'time'.

It should look something like this:

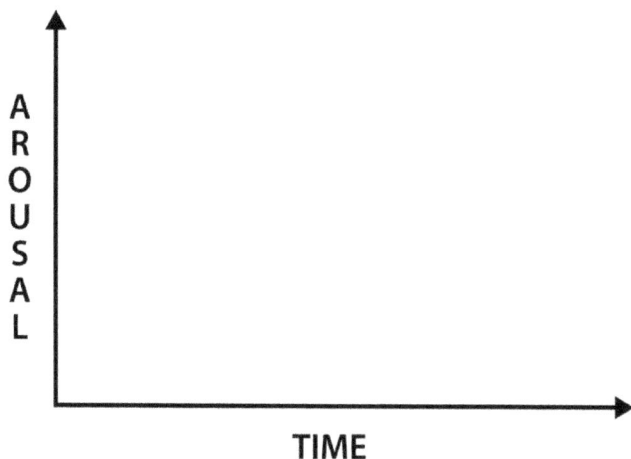

This graph is going to represent how much time we need for our arousal and pleasure to kick-in, once we've started touching and playing either with ourselves or a partner. We're tracking our arousal response. As you move to the right, this indicates time passing. As you move upwards, this indicates your level of arousal increasing.

Imagine now, that you're getting sexy with yourself or a partner. This is where we're at the very start of the graph, where X & Y connect at the bottom left. I want you to draw a line on this graph, starting at this point, that shows what you feel your current arousal response is over time. You could get specific with this if you like, but mostly, let's just use this broadly as a guide and note that this graph could represent around an hour of time.

To repeat the task, imagine you're getting intimate with yourself or a partner. I want you to draw on the graph, a line representing what you think your arousal and pleasure response is like over time.

Here's an example of what this *could* look like:

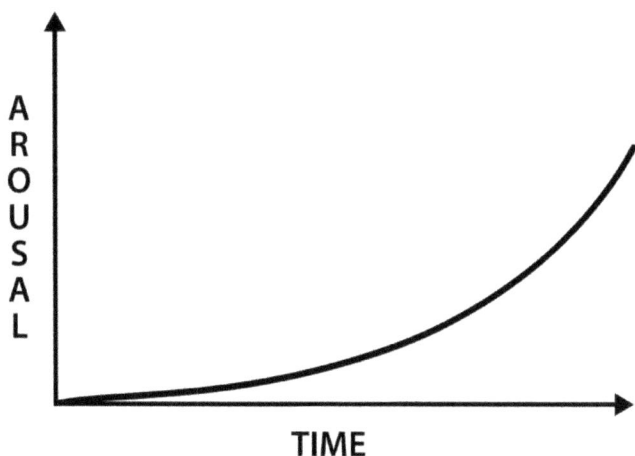

This graph shows that this person doesn't have an immediate arousal response (which is very normal), however after some time and a bit of lovin, they start to enjoy things more.

Now, if you're currently doing this with another person, I'd like for you to draw a second graph, and on this one, you're going to redraw your own line on it, and also in the same graph in another colour, copy this other person's line into it also. Then, circle where those lines intersect (if they do). So, you have two (or maybe more if you're with multiple people) lines on the one graph, giving us a comparison.

It *could* look something like this:

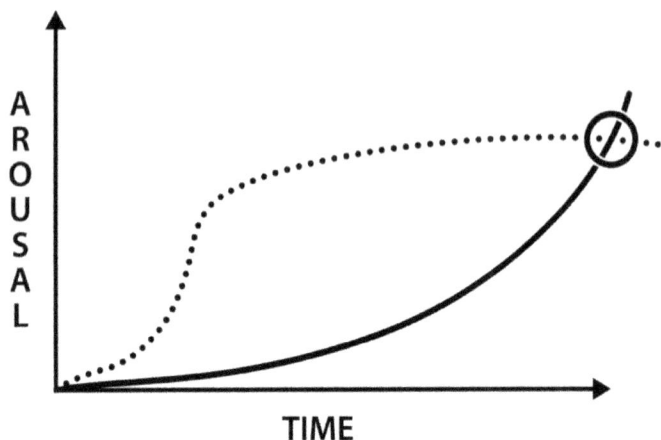

For many people the lines vary quite a bit and for others, not so much. There's no right or wrong here, we're simply visualising the invisible processes within our body. No matter how similar or different these lines are, it's extremely rare that the lines would be identical.

Why? Because we are all different, as is our sex and our pleasure. But the two parts of this graph I want you to focus on is the part where the lines intersect, and the space in between the lines which I've highlighted on the next graph.

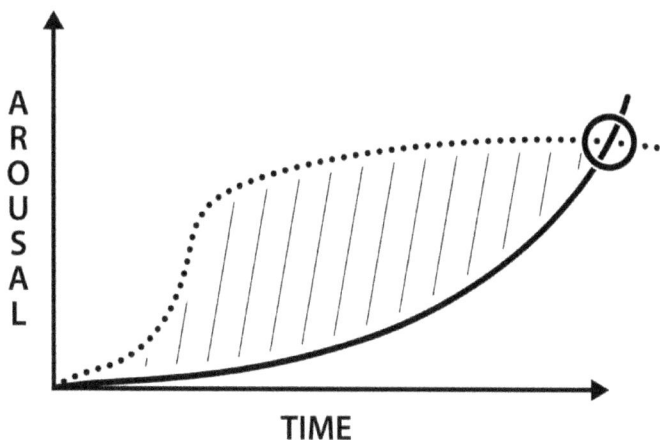

The space in between the lines represents the time in your connection and intimacy, where you're mismatched in your pleasure and arousal. One of you is more aroused, faster. What we want to do is get you to the point where those lines intersect, because this is your happy spot. This is where sex is pleasurable and enjoyable for all involved. This is the sexy goldilocks zone.

That highlighted space is the guide for you to know how much more time and attention one person needs, so you can get to that intersection point for mutual enjoyment. This is fantastic to know, because guess what? If you need more time and attention, we can give you more time and attention!

Brainstorm together, right now, some things you can do together or alone, that will help the person who needs a little more time, to feel relaxed, feel sexy and feel aroused. What things could you do at the start of your play and intimacy that will help this person arrive into their body and pleasure, so you're both on the same page? Is it a massage? A warm bath followed by some soft touch? Is it soft kisses on the neck and lower back? Is it watching some porn together? Use that space in the graph, the mismatch in your pleasure as a guide on how to get your pleasure to match. This is how sex becomes more enjoyable for everyone and ties into the thing that will contribute you to wanting it more. If we're having lovely experiences with ourselves/partners, we will be creating those positive pleasure neurological associations and want it more!

For people doing this individually, look at the curvature of your line/arousal. Is there a lot of time where you aren't feeling pleasure and those arousal responses? Think about your self-pleasure practices. Are they rushed? Do you go straight to the genitals? Do you feel frustration that you're not 'getting there' fast enough or at all? Brainstorm for yourself, are there things you could do to help you drop into your body and its pleasure before you self-pleasure? Erotic dancing, full body touch, porn, erotic literature, what can you integrate into your pleasure practices so you can really connect with your pleasure and arousal?

The next time you're planning a sexy date with yourself or another, remember the graph, your reactive arousal and look at these things you've brainstormed. Plan a few of these at the start of your connection, to give the person who needs a little more time and attention just that. This is how we all have a better experience, this is how we can ensure a pleasurable experience for all, even with a slower arousal response.

This can be tricky for some people, and the idea of receiving more attention than the other may be surprisingly difficult. We're raised in a culture to believe that sex is some form of an exchange. Well, it's not. You don't give, *just* so you can receive. There should be no agenda in sex. If you need to receive more attention, more touch and more focus in sex, please know you're not a selfish lover. You don't need to 'return the favour'. Sex is a gift and doesn't need to be strictly two-way all the time. Remove the agenda, so you can access your pleasure.

If you drew a comparison graph and the multiple lines on it don't intersect, perhaps one of your lines looks almost horizontal, that's okay. That happens and you're definitely not the only one. Please know there is hope. You can rehabilitate your arousal and work towards getting those lines to intersect, towards getting your line to move upwards quicker. How? By neurological sensate activities to enhance and recover pleasure responses via my online libido recovery masterclass 'Connection and Cancer (detailed in the 'resources' section), the 'Penis Pleasure Masterclass' designed for pleasure and erectile recovery (also detailed in the 'resources' section) or refer to some of the information in the 'changes in erection section'.

If you love the idea of intimately playing with each other, touching and reconnecting, but aren't sure how, I will share a list of ideas shortly in the upcoming section 'simple ideas for connecting'. In particular, 'chatty massage', the '2-minute game' and 'active receiving' are worth considering.

Another note on exercise.
A study which was done comparing the impacts of light to moderate exercise in increasing sexual satisfaction, had two

groups. One where people had to go for a quick jog before having a sexual experience and then rating it, versus people that didn't exercise and rated their sexual experience (the sexual experience was everyone watching the same erotic film). Most of the people that went for a jog beforehand had a much greater satisfaction score compared to those that didn't. It wasn't a huge study, but worth mentioning as the results make perfect sense. Exercise gets blood-flow to your pelvis and deeper genital structures, increasing sensitivity, pleasure and tissue engorgement, all the things that make up arousal! If you're able to time your sexy-time after you have some exercise, it may genuinely help quicken and intensify your arousal response time.

Just like when discussing the benefits of exercise and erection recovery, please do not read this as me saying all you need to do is go for a jog and your sex will be perfect. Exercise is something that can help, but is not a cure. It is still important you sit down with yourself and/or your partner and do the above arousal graph and brainstorm together. Going for a brisk walk before touching and getting intimate so you're/you're both on the same page could be the difference between having a good time, and a great time.

6. IT'S TOY TIME!

In this section, I'm going to be discussing a few toys out there. I'll never be able to cover it all as it's endless. So, I'm only going to be chatting about a few *types* of toys that I often recommend to clients, who are experiencing changes in their arousal and pleasure.

Firstly, and most importantly. Toys don't mean something is wrong, toys mean something is right! Think of it, the word 'toy' is perfect. It's about fun, it's about play. Approaching sex with playfulness, exploration and curiosity is how to ensure you have a good time on so many levels.

I'm going to start with vibration, as it's a wonderful tool to use for people that have mismatched desire and delayed arousal, and can be a very useful (and fun) way to get someone into their pleasure quicker.

Vibration

Toys that vibrate have a few main purposes which are to offer heightened stimulation and to access deeper tissues. There are countless types of vibration toys and I'll cover a few, but remember this. Vibration is a wonderful method to offer a type of stimulation to parts of our body that we can no longer stimulate ourselves and also offers stimulation in a way we cannot do naturally or anymore. Plus, vibration is felt *deeper* in the body, so it can be more arousing because it reaches more tissues internally. If we're experiencing numbness or changes in sensation and pleasure, exploring with vibration can be a way to stimulate our arousal, when things aren't working the same as they used to.

There are vibrators for penises, vaginas, anuses, the clitoris and there are so many to choose from.

They can be used at the beginning of play, to kind of kick-start pleasure and arousal. They can be used during play, to maintain arousal or increase pleasure. They can be used at the end of play, if perhaps someone wants to heighten their pleasure in the hopes of reaching climax with another partner, or to 'finish-off'.

Or all of the above.

Vibration can be great for people that have changes in genital sensation and may be experiencing 'numbness' and can be a great way to 'wake up' the sensory receptors.

There is no right or wrong way to use them, as long as

you're exploring and going slowly the first few times you play with them. When our bodies change, so does our sensitivity, so we can 'overload' ourselves if we go too fast too soon.

I'm going to now introduce you to a very popular vibration toy called the 'doxy wand'.

<u>Doxy massager wand:</u>

The original model was a 'Hitachi wand', which is almost identical to the 'doxy wand', known to be one the most intense vibration toys that exist and were originally designed for deep tissue massage. There are many models available including less expensive ones with a slightly less powerful motor (I think if you type in Amazon or eBay 'body massager' you'll find a bunch). These toys are not designed for internal use, but the vibration is so strong you feel it throughout your whole body regardless.

This toy is wonderful when being held against an anus, penis and that magical perineal space between the scrotum and anus. You *must* start slowly, at the lowest setting. If you start at a higher setting you may get overwhelmed. This is also wonderful for massage and if you're getting intimate with a partner and offering sensual touch, pop this out and use it for relaxation. It's amazing on the lower back and shoulders and helps me get through migraines when I use it on my neck.

Tip #1; When you're using it, pop a condom over the head and a few drops of lube. That way when you're done you can simply pull the condom off and give it a wash in soapy warm water and it's perfectly clean. Plus, with the lube it just makes things smoother and more enjoyable (we always want to prevent friction).

Tip #2; You can use this toy through your hand by placing it on the back of your hand while you're touching someone. This is the toy that can magically turn your hand or fingers into a vibrating hand! And yes, it most definitely does feel good (a friend of a friend told me).

Vibrators for penises:

They do exist in varied forms. I will, however, recommend ones that cup around, or somewhat surround the penis, to offer more stimulation and also offer pleasure regardless of how erect you may or may not be. This way, it can be used for both soft or hard penises and offers better stimulation. Remember, vibration is an internal stimulator and can offer people with soft penises incredible pleasure. It's all about exploring. The 'mantra' and the hot-octopuss 'guybrator' are two which seem to make many people happy.

Anal toys

There are so many varieties of anal toys and I could speak on the topic of anal pleasure forever (and do when I'm running anal-pleasure workshops), so I'm going to keep this super brief.

Most people have had a bad anal experience in sex, for various reasons and most people I coach feel that because they didn't enjoy it then, means they don't enjoy it at all. The anus is capable of extreme pleasure, that it needs to be relaxed to be ready (like the rest of our body) for play and penetration. Start with gentle massage, hold some vibration on the outside of the sphincter (like using the doxy wand resting against your finger, so your vibrating fingertip is stimulating the anal entrance), give your body and mind time to relax.

Always start with the smallest toys. Buy the smallest butt-plug and only put the tip in, get used to the sensations.

In the shower when you're washing, give the outside of your anus a few moments of soft curious touch.

Vibrating butt-plugs are *amazing* and are great for getting blood to that area and for having orgasms (without any pressure of being erect). Always start small, start slow, start with curiosity. Bigger is not better, what's good for you is what's best for you.

Strap-ons

Strap-ons are pieces of underwear or step-into harness-type coverings, that go over the hips (and can be super comfortable) that hold a dildo/toy in penis position, so a person can penetrate another with hip-thrusting motions. I promise they look more complicated than they are, and are often just a step-in process like putting on underwear to get them on.

Strap-ons aren't only for people with vulvas, but some are designed for people with penises, who may want to have the 'act' and 'motion' of penetrative sex with others, but are mechanically unable to have/maintain an erection to do so. They commonly have a hollow dildo to comfortably slide the penis into, or a hole/pocket for the penis to sit underneath where the dildo/toy is held in place.

This prevents needing to tuck the penis behind the dildo itself, which would push against the penis with each thrust, causing discomfort.

There is no denying that the person using the strap-on has a different experience, as the dildo/toy itself doesn't have sensory feedback. However, this is still a beautiful way to continue a form of sexual connection and action you have previously enjoyed with your partner/lover, that you feel may be lost due to changes in erection. Strap-ons can keep that sexy connection going, if that style of penetrative sex is meaningful to you. Plus, seeing a partner in their pleasure, being responsible for and giving them pleasure from your thrusty movements is pretty hot and still *very* satisfying for the wearer!

If you have a penis and are interested in exploring strap-ons, please make sure you purchase one that specifies it is designed for people with penises to ensure it's comfortable (and enjoyable!).

The blindfold

Yes, this is a sex toy, as well as an object of daily function. This simple and easily found item is a real game changer.

The blindfold can really help quiet that brain-chatter by removing visible distractions and is great to help calm our mind when we're anxious or self-conscious. Plus, when we remove one of our senses, all of the others get heightened. Touch just gets better with a blindfold on. Through decreasing distraction and increasing your sensitivity, this can be a great way to find those erogenous and pleasure zones you never thought existed for greater pleasure. I highly recommend.

Things to consider when buying a toy

Shape. Can you hold it? Is it a shape you could use in your hands (too small, too thin, too large, too wide)?

Buttons. Are the buttons on it large enough for you to use? If you have arthritis or peripheral neuropathy, you may want to choose a toy where the buttons are on the larger side.

Sound. Does it use a motor and if so, does it mention intensity of sound? I often look for toy descriptors that mention things like 'whisper quiet'. If you live in a tiny apartment like I do, I have to consider my neighbours. I always look for 'quieter' toys.

Collaborative. Could a partner or date use the toy on you also? Not a necessity, but does mix things up and creates other levels of fun!

Solo. Can you use this toy on yourself? If you're a bit nervous and new to intimacy aids, going slow and trying it gently on yourself a few times alone can be wonderful if you want to enjoy it with others.

Disability. If you have impaired upper limb function, does this toy come in a box with lots of packaging, have small tiny cable inserts to charge, does it need to be taken apart and put back together again to be cleaned, or is it functional only through pushing small buttons? There aren't many intimacy aids out there for people with limited hand function, so I want to specifically mention the 'Bump'n joystick' and 'the Ziggy' by LUDDI. These toys were both designed by people with disability and healthcare clinicians, the 'Bump'n' specifically for folks with impacted upper limb and hand movement (see the 'resources' section for more info). They're amazing.

So, we've covered some basics in what is an endless topic. Remember, toys are exactly that, toys. They are fun! But also have a lot of benefits post cancer diagnosis as mentioned previously.

If you're not sure where to start, google 'online sex toy store (and your city/country name)'. You will find some.

Check posting to your country, read the reviews online and if they have it available, watch any short videos on how to use the toy.

The international online toy store 'Lovehoney' has lots of 1–2-minute videos on their toys, if you're interested to shop and learn. This can seem a little daunting, but just like everything else in sexuality, approach it with curiosity and exploration, you'll be fine.

7.   UH-OH, WHERE'S MY O?
(CHANGES IN ORGASM)

Something not often spoken about is how during and after cancer treatments your orgasms can change, or sometimes even disappear. This is common (it happened to me and many others I support), this is normal, you are normal.

How can they change, you ask? Maybe they're less 'intense', maybe they're more intense. Perhaps you need a lot more time and play (yum!) to 'get there', maybe your body shakes and does the things it normally does, but you don't really feel any actual orgasm. What I call a *'ghost-gasm'*, and was very strange to me during chemo when I first experienced this. There is also the possibility that orgasms and climaxes may not be possible for a while. Sex can still be very pleasurable during cancer treatments, but sometimes our medications block that 'peak-climactic' experience.

Thanks to the wonders of neuroscience, we now know that our body can 100% relearn how to have them, or have *different* ones.

Firstly, know that there are multiple potential blockers to climaxing. If you're on particular antidepressants or other treatments like chemo, maybe had nerve damage from surgeries and other things, climaxing (orgasms) may not be achievable just yet. It's okay, you can still have a *lot* of pleasure. Sex can still be great sex during and after cancer, without the end point, without that 'goal'.

If you would like to relearn how to have orgasms, or better put, if you would like to rewire your pleasure so the body you now have can have climaxes (even if they're a little different) here's something to try.

Regular self-pleasure with a few rules
I'm talking even just 2-5 minutes a day (10 would be better).

1. Remove the goal, remove the pressure
Ban the orgasm. You heard me! You're only allowed to touch and enjoy your body to rewire your brain and associate touch with *'goal-free'* pleasure. This neurologically starts to rewire your brain in the background that intimacy isn't about the pressure of that goal. This creates freedom and can be a major stepping stone to your pleasure and orgasm recovery. Better yet, if you have a partner/s, have a 'no orgasm allowed' touch-fest a few times a week. Even if

you currently can't orgasm, removing it verbally anyway allows you to enjoy the touch you're receiving (without the guilt, pressure and frustration). Remember, removing the goal can help you get to the goal. You can do this with a partner, but if so, put a timer on and you're only allowed to touch while the timer (5-10mins) is on. It's another way to remove that expectation of it having to 'go somewhere'.

2. Don't forget to breathe

Breath is powerful, as it not only can be used to down or up-regulate our nervous system, but it also aids in circulating blood to our internal tissues. So many of us tense up and hold our breath when we're in pleasure or when we're *trying* to have an intense moment. It's like we're forcing an orgasm to arrive, which is going to get in the way of you having one! It's like trying to force yourself to go to sleep, the effort of forcing it counteracts where you want to go.

Next time you're having pleasure (with yourself or another), relax your muscles and slow down your breath. Remember, this is about pleasure not orgasms, so be curious. Relaxing your body and making sure you're breathing gets blood flow to the deep internal tissues. With blood flow, the tissues get oxygenated and guess what? Our sensitivity increases and so does our pleasure!

If you notice you're tense and/or hold your breath in pleasure, have a few practice runs with yourself. Touch your body, experience pleasure and arousal, but when you notice your muscles tensing up or you're holding your breath, stop, slow down, and only continue when you're relaxed again. Think of it like a pleasure meditation. It can feel strange, but trust me, blood-flow is the key to arousal and pleasure, and we can't circulate blood without breath, and blood can't reach our internal pleasure structures without those muscles being relaxed.

3. Slow it down

Some of my work includes masturbation coaching with clients (refer to the 'Penis Pleasure Masterclass' in the resources section), teaching people that there's more than just fast-paced standard movements. When we rush, we get distracted and then that '*should*' brain (the obligation and pressure of getting somewhere) can get in the way. Plus, as just mentioned, going slow allows blood circulation and muscles to relax... again, blood-flow increases our sensation, arousal and our pleasure. Orgasms may be achievable; they just need more time and 'warm-up'. If this is you, take a look at the 'toys' section, I have some suggestions for you.

4. Massage

A number one way to recover orgasm is through genital massage (refer to the 'Penis Pleasure Masterclass' in the 'resources' section at the end). We all love massage, it's relaxing, allows our muscles to relax and can reduce tightness while increasing blood-flow. Penis massage (preferably soft penis massage) is incredible for orgasm recovery on many levels. Through various massage techniques you can recover and discover new pleasure zones and enhance sensitivity.

5. Repetition

To make change neurologically you need time and repetition. Self-pleasure and/or massage regularly. A few times a week, over months, maybe 5 mins of loving touch every day if you can (but a few times a week if that's more doable for you). Pleasure rewiring is not a quick fix, but from someone who's been-there-done-that after treatments, it can be done!

<u>6. Exercise.</u>

As touched on a few times now (I hope this indicates how important this is!!!), exercise helps with arousal as it gets blood-flow to the deeper pelvis structures, engorging tissues and heightening sensitivity. If you can find even just 10 minutes to go for a quick walk or jog, or do some yoga before a pleasure session, this can not only help recover and improve erectile function, but also increases your sensitivity and arousal, helping pave the way towards orgasms.

<u>7. Lastly, TOYS</u>

Explore with vibration as it offers stimulation to the deeper tissues and in a way we can't offer naturally. It's a great kick-starter for those times when you want to experience pleasure, but aren't sure exactly what your body enjoys. Plus, if you're experiencing changes in erection and/or orgasm, remember that your delightful soft penis is 100% capable of pleasure and orgasms, and penis vibrators that wrap around the shaft can offer intense pleasure without needing to be erect.

Finally, please know there is nothing wrong with using toys. Just like we use glasses to read better, we can use toys to pleasure better. And toy shopping with a partner? Best foreplay ever!

A quick note, that there are some countries which legally sell THC and cannabis products and some folks tell me that specific strains can influence arousal and their ability to climax. I cannot make recommendations as unfortunately Australia is a little behind and it's not legal here, so I can't access this product. I feel it would be irresponsible of me not to mention this, for those who live in countries and specific states of the US that can access this, and may want to look into it further.

This is very general advice and I know our bodies are much more complicated than a few simple steps, but the information here is truly powerful. Our desire and arousal are so complicated during and after cancer treatments, and also for partners. Be kind to yourselves, this is tough and the changes in your body may well be temporary.

8. COMMUNICATING ABOUT SEX

I've mentioned that you will need to be your own sexual advocate, but it really is so important you do ask them.

Why you should ask your health care team?

I'm continually asking you to speak up to your treating team, because if you wait for someone to bring it up, it may not happen. Through an almost complete lack of healthcare professionals initiating a conversation on this topic, I learned that I needed to take the initiative myself to ask the questions. Given how important the topic of intimacy, relationships, sexuality and well-being is, don't be shy - always ask, and if you need to, persist. Medical staff may not voluntarily bring it up, but I've found they are often very well-informed once I ask and are more than happy to have those conversations.

I once asked a nurse while I was in the chemo-chair for advice regarding the ulcers I had on my outer labia. The response I got was calm and not shaming at all, she said she would "ask around" and walked off. She didn't return for over half an hour, so of course I thought she might have been embarrassed and was avoiding the topic, and due to that, I was reluctant to bring it up again. When she eventually returned and didn't mention it, I plucked up some courage and asked her again. The nurse apologised immediately and explained that there was a medical emergency in the next room and it had slipped her mind. She went out to ask the person she was originally going to ask, came back quickly with information, I wrote down the recommendation for a topical cream and everything was fine.

I'm so glad I persisted because my assumption was wrong. The nurse was perfectly happy to discuss it with me, she was just preoccupied with something else. This is a perfect example of how you will need to advocate for yourself and for information about sexuality in clinical settings. Sometimes it's not a priority, but most of the time the staff are so very busy, working tirelessly and these things take a backseat. Another thing that was a pleasant surprise was that the nurses, surgeons, radiologists and pharmacists I spoke to didn't blink an eye when I asked them sexuality-based questions. And they were more than happy to contact the relevant medical professional to answer any questions when they weren't sure what recommendations to give. Medical professionals are trained to talk about bodies, bodily functions and intimate things as part of their job, so, be confident that all you need is to pluck up the courage to ask.

If you do come across a health professional who is uncomfortable when you ask a question or bring up the topic, my suggestion is not to take this personally and just ask someone else, or ask that person who else you could speak with. We've all been brought up with shame around sex and for some healthcare professionals, despite their values and training, might still feel embarrassed. This doesn't have anything to do with you, so please don't take it as a reason to not ask others. You'll find the people around you who are particularly helpful and forthcoming with assistance. I recommend writing their name down so you can focus on directing any questions to them.

Communicating with your partners

Pop-quiz, what am I?

We're not supposed to talk about it, you can't have too much of it, you can't have too little of it, it's used in nearly all marketing to sell but it's never presented accurately in the media, it's a part of human life, social media platforms shut you down for talking about it, people who are different, unwell, older, living with disability, are of different cultures and ethnicities are assumed to not have it or to want it, we receive no education on it yet we're supposed to magically be good at it and we're supposed to always want it....... Yup. That'd be sex.

You may feel from reading the above that you can't win, and sure, our culture doesn't exactly embrace open communication regarding sexuality, but reading this book is how you will learn.

In my experience as a sexuality educator (as well as from my own life), people who are able to talk between themselves about sex more openly, have much better sex. Why, you ask? Because communicating about how you're feeling and what you might enjoy, allows you to engage comfortably and pleasurably. It can also reduce feeling like you're forcing yourself, forcing someone else, or causing any possible harm. It's okay if things have changed, our bodies and pleasure always will. If we can learn how to communicate about what we do or don't want, things will be better. Remember, hand holding, eye contact, cuddles, snuggles on the couch, foot/body/hand massage, genital massage, oral genital play, assisting/giving masturbation, self-touch together, watching pornography together or reading erotic literature together, all of these things are sex and all of them are connective.

I'm going to share a story of someone who wrote about their experience of sex after having their penis removed due to cancer. Post-surgery, he and his wife still have regular sex and are even more satisfied with the quality of their intimacy than before. He shared that before cancer he would ejaculate every time they had sex, which would last around 15 minutes. Now, he has orgasms from his nipples, thighs and scrotum being touched (how amazing is the neuroplasticity of pleasure!). He also now offers his wife many more orgasms and their sex lasts on average an hour. He refers to it as more "quality". They communicate more, explore each other's bodies more and pleasure each other more.

A changed body doesn't necessarily mean worse sex or the end of it all together, change can have its rewards.

9. SIMPLE IDEAS FOR CONNECTING

I keep saying connection is possible even with a changed body, but *how* is connection possible? Below I've listed and described some activities that I've taught, read about and love to do - and are my top picks for you to try yourself. These are particularly wonderful ways to be intimate when our bodies are changing or perhaps working a little differently, and the ways we would typically be intimate might not be possible in that moment. It's not an exhaustive list, but will give you a start (i.e., trust yourself and you can decide what works for you). Not all will appeal to you, that is fine. They are varied enough so that hopefully there's something for everyone that seems appropriate to try.

Remember, these can be done to the level that is right for you, with the person that is right for you. These can be done with a close friend, your carer, by yourself, partners and even family members! It's time to *really* connect. Here's a few ways to do this.

Q&A

I am obsessed with this verbal game and full credit to

Roger Butler from Curious Creatures who created it. It's so useful and fun to play if you're in a position where you want to communicate with someone, but it's hard to bring up an awkward topic or start a conversation. It's also great to play any time anywhere, and I love it in social or private settings. It's so simple yet an incredible way to deeply communicate and connect with strangers, loved ones, friends and everyone else. During many of my treatments, I struggled (and still do) to keep up with conversations that involved more than two people as the brain-fog/cancer-brain had my attention span so low. So, I often played Q&A as a way to be able to listen to one person at a time, and still have valuable, connective conversations with the people around me. I also play it one-on-one to have meaningful conversations with a partner or friend, while communicating was/is so difficult. Simply put, Q&A makes good conversation great, and when you're struggling, it's a life-saver.

How it works.

Someone asks a question, any question, such as: How was your day? How are you feeling in your body? What do you love about your partner right now? What is your relationship to your sex? Do you like cake more than ice-cream? Anything.

The person sitting to the left of the person who asked the question, answers it first. When they are finished, it goes to the next person to the left, finishing with the person that asked it.

There are a few extra rules:

- Every answer is perfect.
- Every question is perfect.
- No interrupting someone's answer, wait until they have told you they are finished answering, before sharing your thoughts.
- You can 'pass' on a question (or make something up!).
- You can call 'Tangent' or 'Time' by making a 'T' symbol with your hands. This indicates that someone may be off on a tangent or taking too much time to answer. We always say "thank you" for a 'T'.
- The person who asks the question, always answers it last.

It may seem strange, having a verbal Q&A game in a book about connection and the importance of intimacy, but there's a theme here. Cancer interrupts life, which includes relationships. Medications, fatigue, nausea, stress, it all interferes and open communication for some can seem too hard. Try this game, try it a few times, it was and still is, a 'go-to' for me, when I want to connect.

Where? You can play it anywhere. Try it in the bath, the couch, at dinner, in the car, a BBQ or a few rounds at the end of the week to see how you're going. It's a beautiful time to be honest, because the rules are that you can't be interrupted and every answer is perfect.

This is also your saving grace if conversations are hard, paying attention is tricky and keeping up with multiple people talking at once. If you let people know what you need and where you're at, they will most likely help you out. I noticed social chatter was a way for people to let me know that 'everything was fine'. But it wasn't, I couldn't concentrate, I couldn't follow the conversation, I quickly forgot what people were saying and I got super stressed. As soon as I mentioned I needed conversation to slow down, that's exactly what happened. Remember, you will need to let people know what you need, and they will be grateful for the guidance. Q&A is a brilliant way to have social structure, and still offer wonderful connections with everyone present.

Little, lovely treats

Sit down and write a list of 5 - 10 things that are small and easy to do, that make you feel special or connected to yourself. Little, lovely treats. If you have a close friend or loved one, get them to do the same, write a list of little lovely things they enjoy. This could be a foot massage, a bath, a favourite wine, a nice cheese with salami and a childhood film (my personal favourite), moisturising each other's hands/backs/necks/chests, looking at photos together, a blindfolded touch experience, a game of loving Q&A (just described in this section) or dancing to your favourite music.

So, when a time comes, when you're feeling like you would like to connect, be intimate, share affection and don't know what to do? Get the list out and see what you're/you're all in the mood for.

All of these small treats should ideally be things that can be done in your home or very close to where you're staying, and don't take a lot of energy. You want your energy to be spent on connecting and enjoying yourself and others' company, not setting up or travelling to a location.

These 'small treats' lists are your go-to. When you're stuck in your head or having a bad day, get the list out. Soak your feet and moisturise them, do yoga, have a self-pleasure session or pleasure a partner, eat an entire pizza when those taste-buds are back online or get your favourite film and a pot of your favourite tea. The point is that you want an easy way to feel special involving yourself, and possibly those close to you. Simple, sensual, special treats that connect you with yourself/others.

Warming and calming

This small yet intimate task can really let you relax, unwind and get connected. A gentle, beautiful way to connect with yourself or with someone else, is by enjoying a warm bath. Relaxing in a body of warm water (not too hot!) has so many positive effects on the body. Muscles relax, our nervous system down-regulates (relaxes), it can reduce stress, muscle tension eases, pain can lessen, blood circulation improves, the list goes on. Add a cup of tea, a glass of wine, something playing on a screen you can see or some quality Q&A (again see earlier in this section) if you have a 'bath-buddy' with you.

The waterless bath

Baths not your thing, or you don't have one? I have for you, the waterless bath experience. Pop your electric blanket on a nice low setting or warm up a heat pack on the couch and create a warm snuggly cocoon for yourself or for you and your pet, child, friend or lover. The intent is to create warmth, intimacy, safety and connection - baths are not essential for this, but feeling safe and snuggly is.

A royal bathing

Credit for this idea goes to my primary carer, who 'softens' the daily activities to connect and show love, and has also used this technique when caring for a friend while undergoing treatments for brain cancer (spoiler, they loved it!). Is your partner, lover, friend or carer helping you with your personal care? Such as dressing, washing or even simply helping you dry your feet after the shower? If this is the case, every once in a while, ask the person assisting with your care to take their time with it. Turn it into an almost worshipping, lovingly sensual dressing or bathing. Imagine the treatment someone might get in a luxury ancient

Roman spa.

Slowly wash the feet, slowly caress and wash the back, take your time enjoying putting clothing on someone, let the materials softly brush over the skin. Attention and intention are drivers of pleasure and going slowly allows this to happen. Yes, we are often time poor and we go into 'automatic mode', however this is a lovely five-minute task which can be added into daily life quite easily and shows care, love and affection. This small activity acts as a reminder to each other, you're not in a clinical environment, you're not a nurse going through the rounds with a patient, you're caring for someone, someone you care about. Be soft, be gentle, be present. What a treat and what a connector. And it only needs to take an extra five minutes or so.

A simple good night kiss

Life is hectic and a cancer diagnosis doesn't lighten the load. Finances, appointments, family life, medications, symptoms and more, can fill up the days. The only time you may actually see a partner or lover is at the end of the day. If this is you, think about taking five minutes, when you're in bed together getting ready for sleep. Lie down facing each other and look into each other's eyes. Touch noses if you like, hold hands, intertwine feet, hold eye contact, share a good-night statement, breathe together or share a kiss on the lips. It's a time where you're both settling down and both in the same spot, it's a great time to use it to connect.

Don't go to bed at the same time as the person you live/share space with? That's okay, ask that you get 'tucked-in' or tuck your partner in. Get the blankets up to their chin, wish them good night, give them a kiss and a few words of love. It's just such a sweet thing. And if you don't share a house with your loved ones? Sweet, loving good night text messages mean the world!

Self-pleasure

Our entire bodies are capable of pleasure and giving yourself some time, some touch and love is a beautiful way to connect with yourself and get those happy chemicals flowing. During treatments you may be tired, stressed, sore, in pain or feeling flat. Whether you're single or partnered, a lovely way to calm and connect with yourself is to give your body, soft, loving touch. This can, but doesn't necessarily need to involve your genitals or you getting aroused. Our bodies are complicated things and treatments can make our body almost feel like a stranger, so getting to know it again can be wonderful, and is a wonderful way to begin the neurological process of recovering erection.

Give yourself some time, show yourself you're special and set yourself a date. Be it once a fortnight, once a week, or whenever you feel slightly motivated. It's nice, the first few times if you try to leave genitals out of it, just to see what it's like to focus on your body in a different way. We don't give ourselves enough one-on-one time and this is most definitely the case for personal intimate touch. Be curious, explore, hug yourself, scratch, tap, softly touch the skin, find what your body is and isn't enjoying, what it does and doesn't enjoy at that moment. I'm a firm believer that offering ourselves self-pleasure and understanding our bodies is essential for us to be able to connect with others. Regardless if you're partnered or not, having some time with yourself is healthy, it's calming, and it's connecting.

Massage swaps

This may seem like a strange thing to recommend in regards to intimacy and pleasure, but hear me out. Touch, care, love and affection are all things many of us forget about during and after treatments. If you're unsure of what your body wants in an arousal, erotic sense, your immediate fallback plan can be massage. Having someone massage you, gives focus on physical, attentive touch without that pressure of it needing to lead to sex. It's pleasurable, it's intimate and gets you connected (and it feels so good!). Massage swaps can also act as an 'ice-breaker', if you're with a partner or on a date and it's been a while since you've touched each other (which is common). This is a lovely and accessible way to ease back into a physical and touch based dynamic without the pressure to 'perform' or 'be sexy'. If you're not partnered and want some touch, but aren't sure how? There are many very skilled professional massage therapists out there, even the 'pop-in' 10-minute massage parlours have amazing touch and anything that connects you to your body and feels good, is a win.

Another amazing benefit of doing massage swaps, is it's a way for a partner or lover to get used to touching your changed body. So often, I support partners through their fear and anxiety of hurting their partner by touching them. A simple massage can be a way to have your partner touch your body and even start to explore areas they are hesitant to touch (like surgery sites or scars). With a little encouragement, direction and permission from you, these fears and anxieties can be overcome, together.

An undressing ritual

One of the top three most common themes I support people through regarding sexuality and cancer treatments, is changes in body image. And when our sexual function changes, so does the relationship and attitude to our body. How we see ourselves and also, the fear of being naked in front of another person (and/or yourself).

Undressing rituals are a method of removing clothing for yourself, or another, in a way that is gentle while allowing space for nervousness and shyness, while inviting acceptance and positive regard. You can do this solo by yourself in front of a mirror as a way to get used to your new body, or with a date or partners.

How it works.

There's a lot of scope for variety here so feel free to bend and change this to suit you, but here's the basics. Standing in front of the mirror or someone else, you choose one item of clothing at a time to take off, and as you remove it you make a personal statement. Something that is true, that is how you feel, but also as a way to process, release and move towards acceptance. It's a neat psychological trick and can be wonderful. If you're doing this with a partner, take turns, so after you remove an item of clothing and make a statement, they do the same. Then it's your turn again, and so on.

<u>By statements I mean things like;</u>

- As I remove my shoe, I let go of how hard I am on myself.
- As I take off my shirt, I let go of my self-consciousness.
- Removing my belt is me removing the restrictions of society's ridiculous beauty standards.
- As I remove my underwear, I welcome in love and acceptance of my body.
- As I take off my scarf, I release my fear.
- By taking off my pants, I am freeing myself of anxiety.
- By removing my pink sparkly cowboy hat, I am letting go of my tiring day.

Or, if that form of statement doesn't feel right, you could try positive words as you remove clothing and show parts of your body:

- As I look at my arm, I notice the smooth skin I have.

- While looking into the mirror, I'm loving the freckles I have on my face.

- With my chest exposed I feel an appreciation for being alive.

- As I look at my genitals, I notice the awesome curls in my pubic hair.

- As I see my stomach, I see scars/marks of me living, and making it through

- While looking at my lower back, I like the curve where it joins my bottom.

I have done this by myself in front of a mirror, with a long-term partner and also on a date. It was surprisingly effective on the date, as I was very self-conscious about my body and didn't know how to transition from clothed to well, not-clothed. We both took turns slowly removing an item of clothing, we looked into each-other's eyes, we were honest and it was magic. It helped me relax and it helped them understand how I was feeling and how I was struggling.

Go slow. If you're doing this alone in front of the

mirror, it can be quite confronting. Don't feel like you need to fully undress, you may need to do this gradually over time. You could remove one additional item of clothing in the mirror to look at and love each time you do this, so it's nice and slow. I've done it several times alone, as a way to slowly look at myself and get used to my changed and abnormal body. I cried a lot, but it truly helped me with body acceptance and processing my grief for the body I used to have. Follow yourself, breathe and trust that you can stop if you need to.

If you're with someone and you don't want to get naked, you can remove 'imaginary' items of clothing (like an orange feather boa, a sequin vest, rainbow suspenders etc.) or simply ask to stop. You could also do this with someone, where you take turns in removing an item of clothing off of the other person, while making positive statements about their body. Or maybe you choose the item of clothing on yourself to remove and your partner/date shares statements of love and appreciation of that particular body part. The best part of this activity is that there's room to change this to what feels right for you, at the pace that's right for you.

Chatty-massage

If you're liking the ideas in this book about communicating more about what you want and giving more feedback in intimacy and pleasure, but aren't really sure how to do that, this one's for you. 'Chatty massage' is very simple, and is the perfect way to get better at figuring out what you want or don't want, and also, how to ask for it. Plus, this is another excellent activity to do, if your partner is feeling a little hesitant to touch your body.

<u>How it works.</u>

Easiest done in pairs, one of you is the 'masseuse', and the other receives the 'massage'. But there's a twist. The person lying down, the one receiving the 'massage' is actually directing the masseuse on what to do. Sounds easy right? Well, there's a little more to it.

The person who is receiving direction, the 'masseuse' is only able to do exactly that, receive and follow directions. They cannot take over the experience or offer what they *think* the person receiving might enjoy. They can only follow the directions given by the person lying down who is 'receiving' the massage. The most important part of this however, is that if the masseuse/person following directions doesn't hear something along the lines of "keep going" or "I like this continue please" or a new instruction, they must stop touching the person giving the directions all together by gently removing their hands and waiting for the next instruction.

Why does the person have to stop touching after 10 seconds of silence you ask? For the person who is receiving the directions, this is a lesson in being guided in touch, in taking feedback and more importantly, not making assumptions as to what the other person may want and 'winging it'. For the person receiving the massage/giving directions, it allows them to learn how to ask for what they'd like and how to communicate if they'd like something to stop, continue or to change. It's powerful stuff. It's also an incredible way for them to really explore their body and to learn what they do and don't like at the pace that's right for them.

Giving feedback and knowing how to receive it during intimacy is the thing that makes a good time, a great time. But we're not taught how to talk about sex or our bodies. We're definitely not taught how to explore our likes and dislikes in a safe and compassionate way. The world would be better if we were. Chatty massage (as simple as it seems) is your way to flex those communication muscles and learn so much about your and your partner's pleasure.

If you're not sure where to start, try doing it together sitting on the couch and just on the hand or shoulders to start with. Or have a clothes-on play together while you get used to how it works. You could even set a timer so you have 5 or 10 minutes each of giving and receiving while you're trying it out. You can start by exploring things like soft touch on your arms, maybe scratchy touch on your back, massage touch on your neck and thighs. Soft kisses on your lower back. Feel free to get creative as the person following directions is going to stop if you don't ask for it to keep going, or ask for something to change. This is the safety mechanism, so you both can feel free to relax and have a bit of fun with it.

You may be thinking that the more difficult role in this is the person who's lying down and giving the directions. Funnily enough, when I work with partners together and I teach them this activity it's the complete opposite. It's the person receiving directions and having to stop and withdraw touch after 10 seconds of silence that struggles the most! Due to this, I'm going to repeat the rule as it's surprisingly tough for people, but is so important. If the 'masseuse' doesn't hear a direction after 10 seconds, they must stop what they're doing, remove their hands and wait. This is what will help the person giving direction do exactly that, as they will *have* to give you direction when you stop. So much of our intimacy is guess-work and with the impacts of cancer treatments, clarity and communication could never be more important. Stopping the touch after a short amount of time is a way to help each other practice giving and receiving feedback and most importantly, tuning in to what you do and don't want at the time.

It will 100% feel clunky and awkward at first, just like everything else we try in life for the first time. Don't worry too much about it as this is play, and yes play can be clunky, but it can also be fun. Have a laugh and have another go. Communication is the number one sex move, and this activity is the perfect way to practice.

The two-minute game

Finally, we learn about the two-minute game! Life coach Harry Faddis created the 'three-minute game' and I was taught the 'two-minute game' from Roger Butler at Curious Creatures, and it's simply brilliant. This game is suitable for those experiencing treatment and their loved ones, is great when you have no idea how to connect with someone or where to start and is a wonderful way to gently get to know each other's bodies again.

Here's the rules.

- Set a timer or an alarm on your phone for two minutes.
- Pick who goes first, then that person asks for something they would like for 2 minutes (some examples are listed shortly).
- If you all agree, start the timer and give the person whatever they asked for.
- When the timer goes off, completely stop what you're doing.
- Then it's the next person's turn to ask for something they would like for two minutes.
- If everyone agrees, start the timer and go.
- Once the timer goes off, again, stop what you're doing.
- And repeat.

That's it. Really, that is the game. So simple, yet so

effective. You can play it for as long as you like - 10 minutes or an hour, or however long you have energy and are having fun. Time can really fly when playing this game.

Also, this game can be played with anyone, not just someone you're in a relationship with. It could be a friend, family member, carer and doesn't have to be in pairs. There are so many ways to connect, to touch and be touched, which this game can help you discover.

One of the first (out of possibly hundreds) times I played this, I wasn't sure what to ask for. So, of course, I asked for a shoulder massage. Then, that became a slow back scratch. Then full body soft touch and I was amazed at how starting simply and being left wanting more (thanks to that timer) guided me to what I would like next. Asking for what you want can be difficult at first, but this game allows you to develop that skill with practice. Asking for what we want is such an essential skill to have during cancer treatments (and always).

A common question when introducing the two-minute game in workshops is, "what happens if someone asks for something you don't want to do?" Say "no-thank you" with a smile and discuss an alternative (such as touching the chest or back rather than genitals). It's okay. Wait, it's more than okay, it's wonderful to say 'no'. Saying what we don't want is equally (maybe more) important than saying what we do want. The goal is to find that optimal place where everyone is happy giving and receiving.

<u>Here's a few reasons why this game can work for you:</u>
Our genitals aren't always up for being played with, so when it's your two minutes, ask for something that doesn't include them (you have your whole body).

This game can allow connection, even with different levels of libido. Someone might want sexual touch for two minutes and if you're happy to give it, great! Your two minutes could be something that suits your mood such as "tell me your favourite joke using your hand as a puppet". The possibilities are endless and you can ask for exactly what you want, while easily avoiding what you don't want.

Bodies impacted by treatment can change dramatically and unpredictably, be it sensation, arousal, pain, surgical sites etc. This game allows you to relearn how your body works or doesn't work (where those desensitised parts are, where it's sore, where it's pleasurable, how toys or lubes feel).

If you're playing this with a partner and are worried

about where things may lead to? Take 'typical' sex off the table for the entire game. You could have a 'no genital contact' rule or even leave your clothes on. Remove the pressure to perform or get aroused. Obligation & expectation are the enemy of arousal, feeling safe and relaxed is its catalyst. Get creative, enjoy yourselves without that pressure. You can enjoy pleasure from soft intimate touch anywhere on the body.

The two-minute game has many communication benefits and can act as a gentle ice breaker. With changed sexuality and changed intimacy (with or without illness), can come distance and avoidance. Talking about sex is not easy, especially when things are different. This game gently offers a way to help navigate those tricky feelings while also acknowledging the elephant in the room. While we're at it, let's erase any feelings of 'being selfish' or 'a taker'. Asking for your neck to be gently kissed for two minutes, or to be told why this person loves you for two minutes, is simply playing the game. It can seem difficult, but remember, you have to ask, it's the rules! Through my work as a sexuality and consent workshop facilitator, I'm always shocked at how many people tell me that they have never asked for what they want before. Practice makes perfect and it does get easier the more you do it.

<u>Here's a list of things you could ask for, for your two minutes:</u>

- Can you please lower the lights, put some relaxing music on that I would like, bring me water and join me on the couch in two minutes?
- Hold my hand and tell me how you're doing for two minutes.
- Massage my (insert body part here) for two minutes.
- Starting at my neck, ever so softly touch my entire body, back to feet over two minutes.
- Tell me about your day through interpretive dance.
- Put on a song and show me your silliest/favourite dance move.
- Make me a cup of tea in two minutes.
- I would like to cuddle for two minutes.
- I would like to offer you a shoulder massage for two minutes (that's still your two minutes, but if you're not up for being touched, you can touch others. It's all about what YOU want).
- Massage my head.

- I would like to stroke your hair with your head in my lap.

- Lightly touch my beautiful bald head for 2 minutes.

- Gently kiss my neck/chest/thighs/back for two minutes.

- Show me how you like to be kissed, for two minutes.

- Kiss my face and tell me things you love about me for two minutes.

- Softly breathe on my entire body, ending with my genitals for two minutes (YUM!).

If you're thinking, "ugh, whatever Tess. Some of us don't know how to just simply know what you want and ask for it." You're right, I hear you. None of us are taught this, but I have a solution for you. A beautiful baby-step towards the 2-minute game and flexing those 'asking' muscles, is by playing the previous activity 'chatty massage'.

Active receiving

'Active receiving' is a way to connect with a lover/partner to the level that is right for you, when you're not feeling sexy or like having sex and maybe need a little bit more time to get those feelings flowing.

It's a one-way touch experience, and a great way to enjoy touch. I'll explain a little more. There are many expectations and misconceptions in intimate activities, and a super common one is that it should always be a two-way experience. You give and receive pleasure at the same time. Well, this doesn't necessarily always have to be the case, and I offer you a wonderful way to connect in a one-way touch format, very similar to 'chatty massage' mentioned previously. This is wonderful for people with mismatched libido, delayed arousal responses (detailed in the 'reactive versus proactive arousal' section), if someone is not wanting to receive intimate touch or may not know what they want at that moment, but would love to see a partner have pleasure and enjoy themselves.

How it works.

Someone lies/sits down (or is in any comfortable position), asks for what type of touch they want, and constantly directs that person in how they touch them. The other person does exactly what they are being told to do. That's it! It's incredibly fun and accessible.

Imagine the person giving the touch and receiving the

directions has no mind of their own, they are an inanimate object that only responds to commands. For the person following instructions, it can free you from that common brain chatter ("am I doing this right? Are they enjoying this? Are they pretending?"), as you're just doing what you're told.

Some examples of directions the person who is receiving touch (and giving all directions) could give are: "Massage my shoulders. Can you now scratch my back? Yum, thanks, can you go slower and a bit firmer? Softly touch my body up and down, neck to feet with your fingertips and don't stop until I say. Now, lightly pinch my inner thighs. Breathe cool breath on my nipples." Anything you want, just ask.

Unlike in chatty massage where the person following directions stops all together if they don't hear anything after a short while, in 'Active Receiving', the person giving the touch can check in to see if it's how the receiver wants it ("How is this pressure? Would you like me to move my hands faster or slower?") *without* stopping. The person following directions doesn't change anything, doesn't alter any style without being directed. If the person giving touch doesn't receive any directions for a while and isn't sure if this is still what the person receiving still wants? Keep doing what you were last asked to do and ask the question "how could you enjoy this more?"

Similar to chatty massage, this is an incredible skill to learn in the bedroom. Giving directions, asking for what we want, checking in with a lover to get feedback on their level of enjoyment, communicating your desires, all of this leads to better communication and better sex. If you get tired? Simply stop the activity whenever one of you wants. The goal is to enjoy receiving and to enjoy giving. 1 minute, 10 minutes, 20 minutes, it's all perfect.

If you're unsure, give it a go, clothes on, on the couch, using just an arm or hand. Practice following directions, practice giving directions, practice checking in and identifying what you want. There is no goal here, just to have a touch experience, to give or receive pleasure, and enjoy connecting with a partner. It may feel clunky at first, but with practice it flows very easily and you will be amazed at how much you learn about your partner and their body (and yours!).

If this sounds like fun to you, but asking for what you want and giving directions seems a bit daunting, or taking directions and not being the one driving the experience sounds tough, I recommend playing 'chatty massage' or the '2-minute game' a few times first, before jumping into this activity. I say this only because it won't be enjoyable if you're still getting used to these styles of intimate communicating. Those two activities are a wonderful (and fun!) way to develop these amazing sexy skills.

10. TIPS FOR LOVED ONES

Seeing a loved one go through cancer is tough, and so can knowing what to say or how to act. Whether you're a carer, friend, family member or partner, there are ways to offer connection without overstepping a line. And don't worry, we won't break!

It's also normal, when seeing a loved one be so unwell, to want to avoid causing any other harm and through that, create physical distance. That might look like reducing touch and physical contact, or even like possible avoidance. If you're a partner, lover, friend or carer of someone during treatment, I implore you, I beg you, to offer them touch. Treatment is damaging and also detaching. We need the treatment, yes, but we also need care, to feel connected to ourselves and to those around us. Don't be afraid of us, be cautious and curious with us. Think of it as getting into 'ask first' mode.

For simple touch, a peck on the lips or cheek? It's okay! We are not radioactive, we won't give you cancer and we won't break, if we all just take a little care. How do we know what to do or what not to do? We ask.

How to say it out loud.

- "Would you like me to take your hand?"
- "Is there any way you might like some loving/comforting touch right now?"
- "Would you like a hug?"
- "I'd love a cuddle; how does that sound to you?"
- "I'd love to connect with you, are there any sore spots I should avoid if I went in for a cuddle?"
- "I'd love to connect with you right now, is there a form of touch you would like?" (Arm around the shoulder, hand holding, hug from behind, foot massage and more.)
- "I love you and want to offer you affection, is there anything that would comfort you at the moment?"
- "I miss you, but I'm worried I'll hurt you if I squeeze you too hard. Is there a way I can snuggle into you?"
- "I'm wanting to show you love and affection, such as a kiss on the lips or cheek, how do you feel about that?"
- "I'm checking you out right now, fancy a kiss?"

If you're being made an offer of connection and it's not a good time? I offer some examples shortly on ways to navigate that, however a simple, "thank you, but I'm not quite up for it at the moment" is perfect. Even if the person receiving this offer is not up for it right then, you're showing love, care, concern for their well-being and the desire to remain connected. It means the world.

Not in the mood?

Whether you're the person with cancer or the partner of, there will be times when you don't feel like being intimate with others, that is fine, that is normal, that is understandable. There will also be times when you feel like connecting somehow, but aren't sure how. There are lots of places to start: Get in the bath and relax or wrap yourself in blankets with a hot-water bottle, maybe touch your body, snuggle a pet with your favourite film, ask the person you're with to intertwine your legs while you both sit on the couch or lean into their chest. During treatments, you're not going to want intimacy or touch all of the time, so feel free to let loved ones know how you're feeling and speak up in the moments it seems plausible. If you do receive an offer of intimacy and connection and you're not up for it? Remember, that's okay, that's fine, that's normal. But also remember to say thanks for the offer and be kind when you say no thanks, because you want the offers to keep coming!

How to say it out loud.

- "Thank you, that sounds amazing, it's not the best moment, can we see how I'm going later?" (Or tomorrow, or after lunch)
- "Thanks, I'm feeling quite nauseous/tired/some pain, for the moment I need to sit still, can we maybe connect later or another day?"
- "I'm really not feeling well, I'd like to sit alone for a while. Thank you so much for offering a cuddle, rain-check?"
- "I'd love to kiss you, but my mouth is a bit sore at the moment, would you like some soft neck touch instead?"
- "I'd love a hug, thank you, could you be careful around my arm? It's a bit sore."
- "I don't think I'm up for a hug right now, would you like to hold my hand?"
- "I'm pretty low on energy at the moment, but something soft and gentle would be lovely, like a snuggle?"

- Or if you're ADHD and ridiculously blunt like me "Thanks for the offer of a kiss, I'm currently trying not to vomit in my mouth, so will need to rain-check" (we both had a giggle at that).

To those undergoing treatments, if you feel your partner/lover/friend is avoiding you, unattracted to you and doesn't want to touch you? They may just be thinking they are protecting you, avoiding potentially hurting you or feel like they're pestering/pressuring you, so are pulling away. Be the one to communicate and offer a connection. Offer to snuggle, offer to touch their back while they're standing next to you, ask for a long hug hello, it guides them, and can lead to further connections. It meant the world to me, having my hand held and legs entwined on the couch with a cup of tea and chats. It was meaningful and intimate, that at times was my sex. Simple things like that were so important, and I know is/was to others during treatments.

11.   FOR MY FELLOW RAINBOW-FLAGGERS

For people in the LGBTQIA+ community, medical institutions can be very difficult. I remember sitting in the chemo-chair with my then partner holding my hand. The nurse approached and looked at us holding hands, then looking at her said "oh, isn't that sweet you're such good *friends*". I know the nurse meant well, but it was devaluing to me and my partner. I did not feel like I was seen as a person, nor my partner respected. I also did not have the energy to continually educate everyone around me all day every day and advocate for who I am and for others. It's exhausting and with cancer, I didn't have it in me. So, I withdrew and I became reluctant to share my personal story with most clinicians. This is particularly important for people with cancers such as prostate, testicular, cervix, ovaries or breast (just to name a few), as these cancers are *very* gendered. Due to this people can isolate themselves from the supports that are out there as they may feel unwelcome or unseen. Speaking personally, the 'sisterhood' is very strong in breast cancer and as a non-binary person, was difficult to ignore. I avoided so many (pretty much all) support networks due to this as I did not feel welcome. If you're someone who resonates with this, if you belong to communities that are marginalised, I ask you to reach out. Reach out to that one person on your treating team you can have an honest, non-shaming conversation with. Reach out to the nurse asking for any resources the hospital knows of that are accessible and inclusive. Reach out to a friend, to find a cancer support group near you or online that is gender aware, recognises pronouns, alternative relationship models, and partnerships that are not only heterosexual. They are out there, but you may need help finding them. Feeling safe and supported is everything.

RESOURCES

Because there's limited work on sexuality and cancer and well, actual realistic and accessible sexuality education in general, resources can be hard to find. So, here are some, of varied mediums depending on what suits you best.

The 'A Better Normal' mini-book series

Available globally on Amazon in paperback or eBook format, you can search by author 'Tess Devèze' or by book title.

If you're needing support, practical solutions and guidance on more specific side-effects, or looking for help regarding a specific treatment, the 'A Better Normal' mini-book series covers quite a range.

Books in the 'A Better Normal' mini-book series are:

- 'A Better Normal for **Libido**; Your Guide to Rediscovering Intimacy After Cancer'
- 'A Better Normal for **Vaginal Dryness & Pain**; Your Guide to Rediscovering Intimacy After Cancer'
- 'A Better Normal for **Body Confidence**; Your Guide to Rediscovering Intimacy After Cancer'

- 'A Better Normal for **Chemotherapy**; Your Guide to Rediscovering Intimacy After Cancer'
- 'A Better Normal for **Hormone Therapy**; Your Guide to Rediscovering Intimacy After Cancer'
- 'A Better Normal for **Fatigue**; Your Guide to Rediscovering Intimacy After Cancer'
- 'A Better Normal for **Changes in Erection**; Your Guide to Rediscovering Intimacy After Cancer'
- 'A Better Normal for **Radiotherapy**; Your Guide to Rediscovering Intimacy After Cancer'
- 'A Better Normal for **Pain**; Your Guide to Rediscovering Intimacy After Cancer'

The all-in-one resource, 'A Better Normal; Your Guide to Rediscovering Intimacy After Cancer'

Available globally on Amazon in paperback or eBook, you can search via author 'Tess Devèze' or by book title.

If you liked the information in this book, but feel you need guidance on more, the book 'A Better Normal; Your Guide to Rediscovering Intimacy After Cancer' has all of the information included in the entire mini-book series and more. It's your one stop shop for everything you need to know about sexuality and cancer, in the one book.

Penis Pleasure Masterclass

(connectable.podia.com/penis-pleasure)

For anyone with a penis who is experiencing changes in erection and orgasm, or is experiencing loss of sensation, function and pleasure. This online Masterclass teaches soft penis massage, which can be done on yourself or with a partner. Through massage and neurological concepts, things like sensation and pleasure can be recovered while helping recover erectile function through increasing blood-flow with massage. This Masterclass is particularly beneficial for people post prostatectomy.

Vulva Pleasure Masterclass

(connectable.podia.com/vulva-masterclass)

For anyone with a vulva who is experiencing pain and dryness, or is experiencing loss of sensation, pleasure, arousal and orgasm. This online Masterclass teaches vulva massage, which can be done on yourself or with a partner. Through massage and neurological concepts, things like arousal and pleasure can be recovered while helping heal tissues through increasing blood-flow with massage. This Masterclass is also suitable for people with vaginismus and vulvodynia.

A libido and intimacy recovery program for couples
'Connection & Cancer: Reclaim Your Intimacy & Desire'.
(connectable.podia.com/libido-after-cancer)

If you would like personal support of *how* to recover your pleasure, intimacy and libido, then this is for you. It's with me online guiding you every step of the way, and is done in the privacy of your own home. Filled with information, fun and practical solutions that I take you through for libido recovery. The people who I've worked with in this program are having life-changing results. It's an absolute honour to guide people to recover what they felt was lost forever.

'ConnectAble Therapies' (connectabletherapies.com)
For consultations and further resources on sex, intimacy & cancer.

Facebook global support group: *'Intimacy and Cancer'.* This group is for any cancer, any gender and is a very supportive space.

Instagram '@connectable_therapies', where I regularly share helpful information.

YouTube Channel on sex, intimacy & cancer: type *"Intimacy and Cancer CHANNEL"* to find it.

If you prefer video formats over reading (as cancer-brain & reading don't go well together), this YouTube Channel is filled with short videos discussing all things sex, intimacy and cancer.

'ConnectAble Courses' (connectable.podia.com)

A site of intimacy and cancer online courses for sexual recovery. Including the Masterclasses, libido recovery program and webinar mentioned here.

Intimacy & Cancer Information Webinar

(connectable.podia.com/webinar-intimacyaftercancer)

A free information webinar discussing the impacts cancer treatments have on intimacy and sexuality. It has a particular focus on libido and how it can be recovered.

Other amazing resources:

'A Touchy Subject' (atouchysubject.com)

For people with prostate cancer or experiencing changes in erection. Victoria Cullen is *the* person to go to, about sexuality and intimacy post a prostate cancer diagnosis. She also has a YouTube channel and through her website access to free resources and rehabilitation programs.

'The Penis Project' (thepenisproject.org)

This podcast hosted by Sexologist/Nurse Practitioner & Physiotherapist working in erectile and continence health is a wealth of information. Not only through the expertise of Jo and Melissa's (the hosts) clinical expertise, but the personal experiences of the people they interview.

'The Art of The Hook Up' (artofthehookup.com)

This site from dating expert and communication extraordinaire is by Georgie Wolf. Not cancer specific, but incredibly on-point and with relative information for anyone struggling with the dating scene. She has podcasts, blogs, eBooks and more. She's also a workshop facilitator and a bit of a superstar here in Australia!

'Curious Creatures' (curiouscreatures.biz)

For online workshops and much more education on self-development and sexuality. They provide articles, podcasts and streamable workshops which are all very practical and very accessible. I have the privilege to work for this company, their work is changing lives.

'Bump'n Joystick' (getbumpn.com)

An intimacy aid designed for people with impaired upper limb and fine-motor function. Suitable for all genders and is flexible to varied body shapes. This toy was designed by the global disability and OT community, and it's pretty incredible.

'The Ziggy' (luddi.co)

Another intimacy aid designed for people with limited upper limb and intact fine-motor function. Designed by the disability community and healthcare professionals, this is a multi-purpose vibrator for all genders. It's also able to be used while in a wheelchair, so is a wonderfully accessible item.

Pelvic and sexual health osteopath

For those who live in Melbourne, Australia, we have one of the top pelvic health osteopaths you'll ever find. Dr Andrew Carr from the *Whole Being Health Collective'* is referred to as *'the body whisperer'* in clinical and sexual health circles. He works with the entire body, however has expertise and clinical focus on pelvic and sexual health. In particular, people experiencing pelvic pain including after treatments, vaginismus, atrophy and is trauma informed.

If you're not located in Melbourne, there are pelvic floor osteopaths, physiotherapists and OTs all over the world. Simply search online "Pelvic floor osteopath/physio/OT (insert the name of your city/town here)". You'll find someone near you.

Support groups in your area

If you search in google "Cancer Support (insert city/town where you live here)", there should be a list of businesses and companies that have programs near you. Some online or in person. They mightn't be sexuality specific, but there is always opportunity for discussions and learning.

ACKNOWLEDGEMENTS

For anyone and everyone out there affected by cancer, this book is for you. There can be so much to consider, to have to endure, to have to keep track of, that many parts of life take a back seat. Thank you for caring about your intimacy and connections during such a time, be it connections with yourself or with others. I hope you're supported and I truly hope there is something in this book for you.

I'm forever grateful to my clients and the thousands I support online who so openly and vulnerably share their struggles, and also their triumphs with me. This book would not exist without you. I'm inspired and amazed by you all, daily.

Thank you, to my partners and carers over the years Rog, Robi and Kane, my family and my global network of friends. There were some very dark places during treatments and you all got me through. To my booby buddies (my breast care nurses) Claire & Monique, you're my angels. Ricky Dick my oncologist - you're simply the best (Tina Turner style!) and to my RADelaidies.

Lastly, to acknowledge the incredible ethics, values and

approaches to sexuality and communication from Roger Butler at Curious Creatures (and their generosity with sharing their content with me), the occupational therapy & sexuality community (yeah OT-siggers!) and the revolutionary perspectives and therapeutic trainings I received from Deej & Uma, at the Institute of Somatic Sexology (ISS).

ABOUT THE AUTHOR

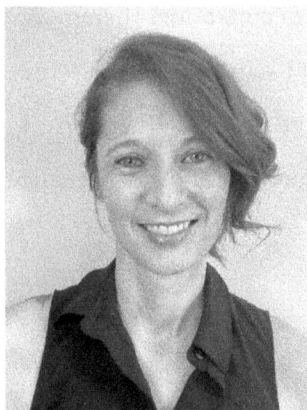

Tess Devèze is an occupational therapist (OT) having completed their bachelor degree in Melbourne Australia, founding ConnectAble Therapies, a community sexuality OT and sexology clinic focussing on sexuality and intimacy for people with neurological conditions, cancer, chronic illness and disability. They have also completed certification and trainings via the Institute of Somatic Sexology. Alongside being a sexuality OT, Tess is also a sexuality educator & workshop facilitator, and has facilitated and educated thousands of people in the topics of communication, consent, sexuality, pleasure and relationship dynamics for nearing a decade. Tess founded the global online initiative 'Intimacy and Cancer', an online support space for people of all cancers and genders to access sexual support.

As a non-binary, queer, disabled person living with cancer, Tess's work is inclusive and advocates for sexual rights for disabled, neurodivergent, gender queer/diverse and LGBTQIA+, communities, which they proudly belong to.

Tess was diagnosed with stage 3 breast cancer at the age of 36 and is still undergoing treatments.

Find them at www.connectabletherapies.com

DID YOU ENJOY THE BOOK?

As an independent author, my work survives through your support. There are so many people affected by cancer, suffering in silence. With each review or word-of-mouth recommendation you make, we can reach the many out there who are struggling and need support.

Please leave a review by visiting where you purchased this book. It's just 1 minute of your time, but could be the thing that helps this reach someone who needs it, someone who needs a better normal too.

Got feedback? Please leave a review! Plus, I'd love to hear from you. You can reach me via email at tess@connectabletherapies.com or via Instagram @connectable_therapies.